GeoSpell French: Spelling Bee Words

There are several thousand words in English that originated in French and are potential spelling bee words. We have identified over 7,000 such words and listed them out in simple and easy format for students to study for local, regional and national spelling bee competitions, held by Scripps National Spelling Bee, North South Foundation and South Asian Spelling Bee.

Words originating from French have a vividly different, and a wide range of pronunciation sounds for many vowels and even consonants. Many of the rules, and some exceptions to those rules, are explained quite well in the Spell It! (www.myspellit.com) by Merriam Webster's, and How To Spell Like A Champ book. We strongly recommend all aspiring spellers to study and understand these rules well

For additional information on these words, such as the definition, part of speech, pronunciation key, etc., look for our book, GeoSpell French Plus.

To the speller: Best wishes for all your upcoming spelling bees! Look forward to seeing you at the Scripps National Spelling Bee. *Study hard, study smart, and study for success!*

Copyright © 2016 GeoSpell Academy, LLC

Title ID: 6405082

ISBN-13: 978-1535150248

Chetan Reddy (2013 Scripps National Spelling Bee Finalist)

Geetha Manku

Vijay Reddy

GeoSpell Academy

Web: www.GeoSpell.com

Email: info@GeoSpell.com

Ph: 214-699-8646

GeoSpell French: Spelling Bee Words

Words from French:

abaisse	accouche	acleidian	adjudication
abandonment	accouchement	acotyledon	adjuration
abatis	accoucheur	acoumeter	adjustment
abattoir	accoutre	acoumetry	adjuvant
abat-voix	accredit	acquest	administratif
abbatial	accumulation	acquiesce	adolescent
abbe	accusable	acquiescence	adonize
abbess	accusant	acrimonious	adret
ablegate	acerb	acrobat	adroit
abri	acescent	acrology	aerobe
abris	acetimeter	acrospore	aeronaut
absidiole	acetimetry	adage	aerostat
absinthe	acetometer	adai	affiche
absinthism	acetometry	adaize	affiliation
abstergent	acetous	adamine	affined
academician	acharnement	adamite	afflux
acajou	Acheulean	adapt	affronte
acceptant	acid	adduction	aggression
accessible	acidifiant	adherence	aggroup
accipitrine	acidity	adhesion	agiotage
acclimate	acidulant	adinole	agneaux
accolade	acier	adive	agnel
accolle	acierage	adjournment	agogue
accommodable	acinous	adjudicataire	agouti

GeoSpell French: Spelling Bee Words

agrafe	alcoholature	allonges	amphibole
agreation	alcoholimeter	allonym	amphibolite
agregation	alcoholmeter	alloyage	amphigene
agrege	alcoholometer	alouatte	amphigory
agreges	alcove	alternat	amphigouri
agremens	alencon	alternats	amusette
agrement	alesan	alterne	anabohitsite
agrements	alette	altruism	anagrammatism
agriculture	aleuromancy	alunite	analcime
aigrette	alevin	alunogen	analogue
aiguiere	algaroth	alveole	anana
aiguille	algerian	amadou	ananas
aiguillette	aligote	amandin	anatase
aileron	alisier	amandine	anchory
ailette	alizari	amassette	ancree
aitch	alkalimeter	amateur	andalusite
ajoure	alkalize	ambatoarinite	andouille
ajourise	alkermes	ambience	anecdote
ala	allantoid	ambrein	aneroid
alaite	allee	ambrette	anfractuous
alalite	allege	ambulance	angelique
alaouite	allemande	amelioration	angevin
albinism	allemontite	amortisseur	angevine
albinoism	allerion	amourette	anglaise
albumose	allonge	ampangabeite	anglesite

GeoSpell French: Spelling Bee Words

Anglophile	antipathic	apropos	areole
animality	antre	apsidiole	areosystyle
anime	aoudad	aptian	ares
anisette	apartment	aquarelle	arete
anisidine	apercu	aquarellist	argental
anisole	aperitif	arabesque	argot
ankaramite	aphanite	arachide	arid
ankaratrite	aphanitism	araeosystyle	ariegite
annalist	apiculture	araguato	aristo
annelid	aplomb	araire	aristocrat
anneloid	aplome	araneology	arithmometer
annuary	apologist	arboricole	arkose
anole	apophyllite	arborize	armagnac
anolis	apozem	arcade	armenite
anomaliped	appanage	arcature	armistice
anomalipod	apparentement	archaeology	armure
anonym	appaume	archaic	arolla
anorthite	append	archducal	aromatherapy
anorthitic	appendicle	archduchess	arquerite
anorthose	apperception	archduchy	arrangement
antagonism	applique	archegone	arrestation
antennule	appreciation	archive	arret
anthoinite	apprise	archlute	arrivism
anthracnose	approbative	archontate	arriviste
anthropometry	apres	ardoise	arrondi

GeoSpell French: Spelling Bee Words

arrondissement	assonant	aurignacian	azarole
arsenate	astucious	aurore	azedarach
arsenide	atacamite	austenite	azote
arseniosiderite	atakapa	auteur	azotic
arsenious	atavism	autobolide	azurite
arsenite	atelier	autoclave	baba
arsenous	aterian	autocrat	babine
arson	athrogenic	automatism	babouche
arteriole	atloid	autoroute	babouvism
artesian	atloidean	auvergnat	babouvist
articulation	attache	aval	baccarat
artisanal	attentat	avalanche	bacchanale
artiste	attentats	avalement	bacchante
ascaricide	attitude	avant	backet
asparagine	attributive	avanturine	bacubert
asphaltene	aubade	aventurine	badian
asphyxy	aubain	aviation	badigeon
aspic	aubepine	aviator	badinage
assemblage	auberge	avid	bagasse
assemble	aubergine	avion	bagasses
assiette	auditive	avocet	bagatelle
assignat	aufait	avodire	baguette
assis	auguste	avoyel	bahut
assise	aulic	axinite	baianism
assonance	aune	ayous	baignoire

GeoSpell French: Spelling Bee Words

bailli	bandeaux	barrandite	battement
bajanism	bandelet	barre	batterie
balafo	bandelette	barremian	battu
balancelle	banderole	barret	battue
balanta	bandlet	barrette	baumier
balante	banlieue	barye	bauxite
balaphon	banquette	barytine	bavardage
balisier	baragouin	baryton	bayonet
ballet	baratte	bascine	bearnaise
ballon	barbaresque	bascule	beaucoup
ballonet	barbastel	basque	beaujolais
ballonne	barbeau	basquine	beaujolaises
ballotade	barbette	bas-relief	beaune
ballotage	barbotine	basset	beaus
ballotte	barcarole	bassine	beaux
ballottement	bardane	basson	beauxite
ballottine	barege	bassoon	becard
balsamina	bariolage	bastille	becasse
balsamine	baritone	batarde	becassine
baluster	barocco	bateleur	bechamel
balustrade	baronne	batiste	becquerelite
bamboula	baroque	baton	becuna
banal	barquette	batonne	becune
banality	barrack	batonnier	bedoui
bandeau	barrage	batrachian	bedouin

GeoSpell French: Spelling Bee Words

beguin	berm	bigarade	bistros
beige	bernardine	bigarreau	bituminous
beignet	berrichon	bigotry	bivoltin
beignets	berthe	bijou	bivoltine
bejan	berthierite	bijouterie	bivoltinism
bejant	bertillonage	bijoux	bivouac
belemnite	bertrandite	bikini	bizarre
belga	betafite	bilboquet	bizarrerie
belle	betise	bile	blague
belleric	betises	biliary	blanc
bengaline	beudantite	billet-doux	blancs
benitier	beurre	billety	blanquette
benzil	bevue	billietite	blase
benzilic	bezantee	billion	bliaut
berceuse	bezique	billon	blindage
berceuses	bibelot	bimanal	bloc
berdache	bibelots	bimanous	blocage
beresovite	biberon	binarism	blond
beret	bibliognost	biniou	blondine
bergamot	bichir	bismuthine	blondinette
bergere	bicorne	bisque	blouse
bergerette	bidactyl	bister	blouson
bergsonism	bidet	bistournage	bobeche
berline	bidonville	bistoury	bobierrite
berloque	bifurcation	bistro	bocage

GeoSpell French: Spelling Bee Words

bocal	bossage	boulonnaises	brabancon
boiserie	bosse	bouquet	brachistochrone
boite	bosset	bouquetiere	brackmard
boleite	bottine	bouquiniste	braconniere
bolide	boucharde	bouquinistes	bradoon
bombarde	bouche	bourdonnee	braies
bombardon	bouchee	bourette	braise
bombe	bouchon	bourgade	brancardier
bombonne	boucle	bourgeoise	brandade
bonbon	boudin	bourgeoisie	brassage
bonbonniere	boudinage	bourguignon	brassard
bondieuserie	boudoir	bourguignonne	brassart
bondon	bouffant	bourree	brasserie
bonduc	bouffon	bourrelet	brazilin
bonhomie	bougie	bourride	brelan
boni	bouillabaisse	bourse	breloque
bonification	bouilli	boussingaultite	bretelle
bonne	bouillon	boutade	breton
bonze	bouillotte	boutique	bretonne
bordelaise	boulangere	bouton	briard
bordereau	boule	boutonneuse	bric-a-brac
bordereaux	boulevard	boutonniere	bricolage
boric	boulevardier	boutons	bricoleur
borne	bouleversement	boutre	bridoon
bornee	boulonnais	bovarism	brie

GeoSpell French: Spelling Bee Words

brigade	bronze-dore	bureaucrat	cabotage
brigadier	brouette	bureaux	cabotinage
brigandage	brouhaha	burelage	cabotinages
brilliant	brouillon	burele	cabriole
brilliantine	brume	burette	cabriolet
brioche	brumous	burgee	cachalot
briolette	brune	burin	cache
briquette	brunet	burlesque	cachectic
brisance	brusque	burnous	cachepot
brise	brusquerie	bust	cacholong
brise-bise	brut	butte	cachou
brise-soleil	brutage	buttgenbachite	cacophony
brisque	bruxellois	butyric	cadastral
brisure	bruyere	buvette	cadastre
brocard	buccaneer	byssolite	cadaveric
brocatelle	buffet	caba	cadaverous
broche	buffoonery	cabal	caddie
brochette	buisson	cabane	cadelle
brochure	bulbel	cabaret	cadet
brodequin	bulbil	cabas	cadre
broderie	bulletin	cabasset	caducity
bromargyrite	buplever	cabassou	cafard
bromic	bure	cabassous	cafe
bromine	bureau	cabernet	cagoulard
bronze	bureaucracy	cabot	cahier

GeoSpell French: Spelling Bee Words

caisson	calvados	candor	caporal
cajole	calvaire	canepin	capot
cajoled	camail	canepins	capote
cajolery	camaraderie	cangue	caprice
calabash	camber	canicule	capsian
calambac	cambist	cannelure	capsule
calambour	camembert	cannetille	capucine
calamine	camion	canonicity	carab
calanque	camionette	canotier	carabineer
calash	camisard	cantal	caracal
calculous	camisole	canteen	caraco
caleche	camouflage	cantharidin	caracoa
caledonite	camouflet	cantonal	caracole
calembour	camoufleur	cantonalism	caracora
calin	campagnol	cantonment	caracore
caliphate	campaign	caoutchouc	carafe
calixtin	canaille	capetian	caramel
calixtine	canalization	capharnaum	carapace
calligraphy	canalize	capillaire	carbine
calmant	canape	capillarity	carbineer
caloricity	canard	capillary	carbon
calorie	cancan	capilotade	carbonize
calorific	candid	capitaine	carbonnade
calotte	candiot	capitalist	cardecu
calque	candiote	capitulant	cardinalate

GeoSpell French: Spelling Bee Words

cardite	carpel	castrametation	celestine
cardon	carrosserie	cataclysm	cellule
cardoon	carrousel	catarinite	cellulite
careenage	carte-lettre	categorematic	cellulose
caress	cartogram	catholicon	celt
caresses	cartography	caulicole	celtist
carignane	cartomancy	caulicoles	celts
carillon	carton	caulicoli	cenacle
carillonneur	cartonnage	caulicolo	cenacles
cariole	cartouche	causality	cendre
carlet	casaque	causerie	cendres
carling	casbah	causeur	cenomanian
carlings	cascade	causeuse	cenotaph
carlovingian	casern	causse	cens
carmagnole	casque	causticity	censitaire
carminative	casquet	cavernicole	censitaires
carmine	casquette	cede	censive
carneau	casse	cedra	censorial
carneaus	casserole	cedrat	centare
carnet	cassette	cedre	centiare
carnotite	cassie	ceinture	centigrade
carolingian	cassis	celadon	centigram
carotid	cassiterite	celebrant	centiliter
carotte	cassolette	celesta	centime
caroubier	cassoulet	celeste	centimeter

GeoSpell French: Spelling Bee Words

centralization	chaine	chansons	chassepot
centralize	chaise	chantage	chasseur
centrifuge	chalcomenite	chantant	chassis
centuple	chalcosine	chantarella	chassises
cepe	chalet	chanterelle	chasuble
ceramicist	chaloupe	chanteur	chateau
ceramist	chalumeau	chanteuse	châteaus
cerargyrite	chalumeaux	chanteuses	chateaux
cercle	chamade	chantilly	chatelaine
cercles	chambertin	chapon	chatelet
cereal	chamoisite	chaptalize	chatellany
cerebral	chamosite	charade	chaton
cerise	chamositic	charades	chatons
ceruleite	champagne	charbon	chatot
cervalet	champagnize	charcuterie	chatoyant
cervelas	champleve	charcutier	chaudfroid
cervelat	chancre	chardonnay	chaudron
cerveliere	chancroid	charentais	chauffeur
cesarolite	chancrous	charentaises	chauffeuse
cessionaire	chandelier	charette	chaussee
ceyssatite	chandelle	charivari	chausses
chablis	channelure	charlotte	chauvinism
chacona	chanson	charolais	chebec
chaconne	chansonnette	charpie	chebule
chagrin	chansonnier	chasse	chechia

GeoSpell French: Spelling Bee Words

chef	chevrotan	cholagogue	chronologist
cheffonier	chez	cholesteric	chronoscopy
chellean	chibouk	cholesterin	chrysene
chemisette	chic	chondrology	chrysopal
cheneau	chicane	choral	chrysoprase
chenet	chicaner	choralist	chute
chenets	chicanery	chordee	chylify
chenevixite	chichi	choree	chymosin
chenille	chiffer	choregraphy	chypre
chenin	chiffon	choreography	cibol
cheval	chiffonade	chose	cicatrizant
cheval-de-frise	chiffonier	chott	ciel
chevalet	chignon	chou	cigala
chevaux-de-frise	chine	choucroute	cigale
chevee	chinoiserie	chouette	cigarette
chevelure	chipolata	choumoellier	ciliary
chevet	chirogale	choux	cilice
cheville	chitin	chowder	cinchonine
chevon	chloral	chrematistics	cinchotine
chevre	chloranthy	chrome	cineast
chevret	chloroform	chromic	cinematheque
chevretin	chlorophane	chronaxia	cinematograph
chevrette	chlorophyll	chronaxie	cinephile
chevrony	chlorous	chronic	cinnamate
chevrotain	chocolatier	chronique	cinq-cents

GeoSpell French: Spelling Bee Words

cinquain	claque	cloche	coelanaglyphic
cipolin	claqueur	clochette	coffret
cipollino	clarain	cloison	cognac
circumvene	clarification	cloisonne	cognatic
cire	clarinet	cloky	coiffeur
cired	clarionet	cloque	coiffeuse
cirque	claudetite	clos	coiffure
ciseaux	clausthalite	cloture	coincidence
cisele	clavecin	clou	coincident
cisjurane	clavelization	cloue	col
cismontane	clavicle	clous	colichemarde
cispadane	clavicor	clubbist	collaborateur
cither	clavier	cluse	collaboration
civet	clechee	coagulable	collaborator
civette	clef	coak	collage
civilite	clefs	cocarde	collaret
civilizable	clementine	coccinic	collectivism
civism	clericalize	coccolite	collegiality
claire	clericature	cocher	colletin
clairon	cliche	cocodette	collibert
clairvoyance	clientele	cocoon	colliquation
clairvoyancy	clinic	cocorico	colliquative
clairvoyant	clinician	cocotte	collusory
clairvoyante	clique	codeine	colmatage
clandestinity	clochard	codicillary	colobin

GeoSpell French: Spelling Bee Words

colonnade	communard	conciergerie	congruism
colonnette	communique	concierges	congruist
colorant	communism	conciliabule	conjuncture
colorist	comparatist	concordat	connexity
colossal	comparator	concours	connivance
colportage	compatibility	condescendence	connive
colporter	compatriot	condrieu	connived
colporteur	compere	condyle	conniving
columbiad	complaisance	conferencier	connoisseur
colza	complaisant	confessant	consanguine
comatose	complementary	confidant	conscientious
comatous	complicity	confidante	conscription
comble	compliment	confident	consecutive
comedienne	compote	confinement	conservatoire
comique	compotier	confiserie	console
commandant	compromis	confit	consoling
commanditaire	comte	confiture	consomme
commandite	comtesse	conformateur	conspue
commemorable	concede	conformator	constatation
commemorative	conceptacle	confortable	constate
commis	conceptacular	confortables	constative
commissionaire	concession	confrerie	consternation
commodatary	concessionaire	confreries	constituent
commode	conche	confrontation	constriction
communal	concierge	conge	consultant

GeoSpell French: Spelling Bee Words

contagiosity	conversive	cordierite	cosmopolitan
conte	convive	cordiform	cosse
contes	convives	cordonnet	cossette
contestant	convulsionary	corfiote	costal
conteur	convulsively	corindon	costume
conteurs	copain	corkite	costumier
contexture	coq	cornetite	cote
contiguity	coque	corniche	cotele
continuant	coquecigrue	cornichon	cotelette
continuator	coquelicot	corps	coterie
contorniates	coquet	corpuscule	cothurn
contorniati	coquetry	corruptibility	cotillion
contorniato	coquette	corsage	cotillon
contortion	coquillage	corsetier	cotte
contour	coquille	corsetiere	cottonade
contourne	coquilles	cortege	couac
contractant	corail	corvette	coucal
contrast	corallin	corymb	couche
contrecoup	coralline	corymbs	couchee
contredanse	corbeau	coryphee	couchette
contrefilet	corbeil	coryphene	coude
contrefort	corde	cosaque	coudiere
contretemps	cordeliere	cosmetology	coueism
convenance	cordelle	cosmographic	couette
convenances	cordiality	cosmographical	cougar

GeoSpell French: Spelling Bee Words

couguar	coussinet	cremone	cromorne
coule	coutil	creole	crookesite
coulee	couture	crepe	croquembouche
couleur	couturier	crepon	croquet
coulibiac	couturiere	cresson	croquette
coulis	couvade	cretin	croquignole
coulisse	couvert	cretinism	croquis
couloir	couverte	cretonne	crosnes
coulommiers	couverture	crevasse	crosse
coumarin	crabier	crevecoeur	crossette
coumarou	cracovienne	crevette	crotale
counterriposte	cramignon	criant	crotonic
coup	cramponnee	crible	croupade
coupage	crapaudine	criminality	croupier
coupe	crapette	criniere	croupon
couped	craquele	crinoline	croustade
coupon	craquelure	criophore	croute
courbaril	cravat	crise	crouton
courbette	crayon	crises	croutons
courge	creche	crochet	cru
courgette	crecy	croise	crucial
courlan	cremant	croissant	crudites
couronne	creme	croissants	crus
courtoisie	cremerie	crokinole	cryosel
couscous	crèmes	crombec	cryptogam

GeoSpell French: Spelling Bee Words

cryptogram	cure	cytophore	dauphine
crystallography	curettage	cytozym	debacle
cubism	curette	cytozyme	debarrass
cubitiere	curietherapy	dacquoise	debat
cubomancy	curite	daguerreotype	debauchee
cuir	cursive	daguerreotypes	debiteuse
cuirassier	cuscousou	daguerreotypy	debouch
cuisine	cusparine	daim	debouche
cuisinier	cutidure	dalles	debouches
cuisiniere	cutiduris	Daltonism	debouchment
cuissard	cuvee	damasse	debouchure
cuivre	cuvette	damnification	debride
culasse	cyanogen	damourite	debridement
culet	cyanometer	dansant	debris
cullet	cyanose	dansants	debut
culotte	cyclical	danseur	debutant
culottes	cyclo	danseurs	debutante
cult	cycloid	danseuse	debuted
cultellation	cymene	danseuses	decagram
cultivable	cymophane	dariole	decalage
cultual	cynism	dartrose	decalcomania
cumara	cypriot	dation	decaliter
cunette	cypriote	daube	decamp
cupel	cystic	daubreeite	decare
cupidon	cystography	dauphin	decastere

GeoSpell French: Spelling Bee Words

decathlon	deglutition	demoiselle	dernier
deciare	degras	demonstrator	derout
decigram	degringolade	denim	derriere
deciliter	dehors	denouement	descloizite
decimeter	deism	density	descort
decisive	deist	dentel	deserter
decistere	dejeuner	dentelle	deshabille
declasse	delafossite	dentil	despotat
decolletage	delaine	dentist	despotate
decollete	delicatesse	denture	despotic
decompose	deloul	departement	despotical
decor	deluxe	departements	despotism
decoupage	demarche	depayse	despotize
decry	demarches	deplorable	dessous
dedans	dementi	deplorableness	dessus
dedit	demiglace	deploy	destinezite
defeatist	demimondain	deployment	desuetude
deference	demimondaine	deportment	detach
defi	demimonde	depot	detache
defiant	demitasse	deracinate	detached
defiantly	demivol	deracinated	detachment
deficit	democrat	derailleur	detail
defis	demode	derailment	detent
degage	demographic	deranged	detente
degenerescence	demography	derangement	detenu

GeoSpell French: Spelling Bee Words

deterge	diaphanie	disabuse	dizain
detergent	diaphragmatic	discography	dizaine
detonation	diastase	discotheque	doctrinaire
detour	diathermanous	disengage	doctrinarian
detraque	dichoree	diseur	doctrinary
detritus	dichroite	diseurs	dogmatism
devant	dietine	diseuse	dogmatize
developpe	digestif	diseuses	doigte
devillite	digitigrade	dishabille	dolerite
devot	diligence	disinfectant	doleritic
devote	dinanderie	disinvolture	dolmen
dewindtite	diopside	disoblige	dolomite
dextrin	diopsidic	disome	dom
dextrine	dioptase	disthene	domaine
dey	diorama	distingue	dome
diabase	diorite	distrait	domiciliar
diablerie	dioritic	distraite	domiciliary
diablotin	diplomacy	disyllabism	domino
diagraph	diplomat	dit	dompt
diallage	dipyre	diversion	donnee
diallagic	directoire	divertisement	donnees
diamante	directorate	divertissement	dormer
diamantiferous	directrice	divinize	dormette
diamantine	dirigisme	divorcee	dormeuse
diaphaneity	dirigiste	dix	dose

GeoSpell French: Spelling Bee Words

dosseret	drap	duvetyn	eclaircissements
dossier	draps	duvetyne	eclat
dot	dressage	dynamic	eclogite
douane	dreyfusard	dynamometer	eclosion
douanes	droitural	dyne	economism
douanier	drolerie	dysodile	ecorche
double	droll	dyspathy	ecossaise
doublette	drollery	dyspepsy	ecrase
doublure	drosometer	eau	ecrevisse
douceur	dualism	eaux	ecru
douche	dubitative	ebauche	ecrus
doucine	ducaton	ebauchoir	ecstasiate
doum	ducatoon	eboulement	ecuelle
douppioni	duchesse	ebrillade	efferent
dourine	dufrenite	ecarte	effleurage
doustioni	dufrenoysite	eccrinology	efflorescence
doux	dumontite	echappe	efflorescent
douzaine	dumortierite	echappee	effluve
douzainier	dune	echelette	effraction
doyen	dupe	echelle	effrontery
doyenne	dupery	echelon	egalitarian
dragee	dupes	echelonment	egalite
dragoon	dupion	echoppe	egality
draisine	dussertite	eclair	eglomise
drame	duvet	eclaircissement	egoism

GeoSpell French: Spelling Bee Words

egoist	embranchment	encorbelment	ensuite
egueiite	embrasure	encore	entablature
elan	embroil	endocarp	entablement
elastique	embryology	endocarpal	entente
electorate	embryotomy	endoderm	ententes
elegant	embryotroph	endogen	entomologic
elegante	embryotrophe	endogenous	entomological
elegantes	embryotrophy	endosperm	entomologist
elegants	embusque	endospermic	entomology
eleidin	emeraude	endospermous	entourage
elinvar	emetine	enface	entracte
elite	emeute	enfilade	entrant
ellagic	emigre	enfleurage	entrechat
email	emigree	engobe	entrecote
emails	empennage	enjambment	entrecotes
embarras	employee	enlevement	entredeux
embarrass	empressement	enlevements	entree
embarrassing	enarme	ennui	entrefer
embarrassment	encastage	ennuye	entremets
emboite	encastre	enoptromancy	entrepot
emboitement	encephalic	enounce	entrepreneur
embonpoint	enchainement	ensemble	entrepreneuse
embouchement	enclave	ensiform	entresol
embouchure	encoignure	ensilage	envelop
embourgeoisement	encolure	ensile	envelope

GeoSpell French: Spelling Bee Words

envisage	epileptic	erotical	escritoire
envisaged	epinard	erotically	eserine
envoi	epinards	erotological	espacement
envoutement	epingle	erotology	espadon
envoûtements	epis	erythrine	espadrille
eolienne	eponge	erythrose	espadrilles
epaule	epopee	escadrille	espagnole
epaulement	eprouvette	escalade	espagnolette
epaulements	epsomite	escalope	espalier
epaulet	epurate	escamotage	esparcet
epauliere	epuration	escapade	espiegle
epee	epure	escargot	espionage
epeeist	equiaxed	escargotiere	esplanade
epi	equilibrist	escargots	espontoon
epicarp	equitable	escarole	esprit
epicondyle	equivoque	escarp	esquimau
epicondylian	erethism	escarpment	esquimaux
epicondylic	erethismic	eschalot	esquisse
epidemic	erg	escharotic	essonite
epidemical	ergot	esclandre	estafette
epidemically	ergotism	esclandres	estaminet
epidote	ergotize	esclavage	estaminets
epigene	ergotized	esconson	estampage
epigramme	ergs	escopette	estampie
epilation	erotic	escort	estoc

GeoSpell French: Spelling Bee Words

estrade	eurygnathism	extradoses	falconry
estragon	eurygnathous	extraordinaire	fameuse
etagere	evacuee	extravagance	familial
etain	evaluation	extrinsic	fanchonette
etalon	evase	exuberance	fanfare
etamine	eventration	fableau	fanfaronade
etatism	eveque	fabliau	fang
etatisme	evocable	fabliaux	fanion
etatismes	evoke	fabricant	fantasque
etatisms	executant	facade	faon
etatist	exercitant	facet	faradism
etchemin	exergue	facette	faradize
ethnography	exfoliative	facilitate	faradizer
etiolate	exhumation	faconne	farandola
etiolated	exhume	facticity	farandole
etiquette	exigible	facultative	farceur
etoile	exode	faham	farceuse
etouffe	exogen	faiblesse	farci
etude	exogenous	faiblesses	farouche
etui	expertise	faience	faroucheness
euclase	exploitation	faille	fascicule
eudist	externs	faineant	fascine
eumolpique	extincteur	faineantise	fastuous
euphony	extradition	faineantises	fatalist
eurygnathic	extrados	falbala	fatigue

GeoSpell French: Spelling Bee Words

fauchard	fetish	filigrain	fleche
faujasite	feuillage	filoselle	flechette
fauteuil	feuille	financier	fleurdelise
fauteuils	feuilles	financiere	fleuret
fauve	feuilleton	fingering	fleurette
fauvism	feuilletonism	fixatif	fleuron
faux	feuilletonist	flacherie	flexibility
fauxbourdon	fez	flachery	flic
febrifuge	fiacre	flacon	flicflac
feculence	fiacres	flageolet	flics
federalize	fiance	flair	flong
federation	fiancee	flajolotite	floraison
feint	fibranne	flambe	florencee
felibre	fibroin	flambeau	flotant
felibrean	fibrous	flambeaux	fluavil
felibres	fibrousness	flambeed	fluid
felicitations	fichu	flamboyant	fluorine
feminize	fief	flamingant	focimeter
fenouillet	figurant	flamingants	focometer
fermeture	figurante	flan	foible
fermiere	figurine	flanconnade	foliar
ferocity	filamentous	flanerie	foliole
ferronniere	filasse	flaneur	foliot
festoon	filature	flaneuse	fonctionnaire
fete	filet	flasque	fond

GeoSpell French: Spelling Bee Words

fondant	foundry	fraser	funiculaire
fondante	fount	fraternize	furtive
fondu	fountaineer	fraze	fusain
fondue	fourberie	frescade	fusarole
fonio	fourchee	fricandeau	fuseau
fontange	fourchette	friedelite	fuseaux
fontionnaires	fourchy	frise	fusee
footy	fourgon	frisee	fuselage
forcat	fourierism	friseur	fusibility
forcene	fourmarierite	frisket	fusible
forchette	fourragere	frisolee	fusilier
format	foyer	frison	fusillade
forme	fraca	frisson	fusionist
formeret	fracas	frisure	fustet
formule	fracases	frivolity	gabarit
fortin	fractal	frondeur	gabionade
fossette	fragmentation	fronton	gadroon
foucauldian	fragrance	frottage	gadrooning
foudroyant	framboise	frotton	gaffe
fouette	francien	froufrou	gaffes
fougade	francolin	frustule	gaga
fougasse	francophone	fuchsine	gaiety
fougere	frangipane	fuliginosity	gaine
foulard	franglais	fumagine	gaiter
foule	frappe	funest	galactose

GeoSpell French: Spelling Bee Words

galant	gambrel	gasogene	gazelle
galante	gambs	gasometer	gazette
galantine	gamin	gastrocoel	gazogene
galatine	gamine	gastronome	gedrite
galere	gaminerie	gastronomic	gelatin
galette	gamme	gastronomical	gelinotte
galimatias	ganache	gastronomically	gelinottes
galipot	gangue	gastronomy	gemmule
gallantry	garage	gateau	gendarme
gallet	garancine	gateaux	gene
gallicanism	garbure	gattine	generalize
gallicism	garcon	gauche	generic
Gallomania	garconniere	gaucherie	genestrole
gallomaniac	garcons	gauffrage	genet
galloon	gardevin	gauffre	genets
gallopade	gardevine	gaufre	genie
galop	gardez	gaufres	genoise
galoubet	gardyloo	gaufrette	genre
galuchat	gargouillade	gaullism	genres
galvanic	garigue	gaullist	geodesic
galvanism	garni	gavage	geognost
galvanize	garrot	gavial	geophone
gamay	garrots	gavialoid	georama
gamb	gasconade	gavotte	georgiadesite
gambade	gasogen	gaylussite	gerbe

GeoSpell French: Spelling Bee Words

gerbil	glacon	goiter	graisse
gerbille	glacons	goitrous	grandiose
germ	gland	goliard	grandiosity
germinal	glandular	gommier	graphology
germon	glauberite	gondolier	graphometry
germons	glissade	goniometry	grappier
gerontocracy	glissader	gonnardite	grasserie
geyserite	glisse	gorgerin	grasseye
gharial	glissile	gothian	grasseyement
gibbon	globule	gouache	graticulation
gibus	globulite	goum	graticule
gigantesque	globulous	goumier	gratin
gigolo	glucose	goundou	gratinate
gigolos	glycerin	gourmet	gratine
gigue	glycose	gout	grattage
gilet	glyptography	gouter	grattoir
girandole	gnome	goutte	gravimeter
girolle	gobemouche	governante	gravure
gisant	gobemouches	goyazite	grebe
gisants	gobinism	grad	grecize
givetian	gobony	grade	greenovite
glace	godet	grades	grege
glacier	goffer	gradin	greige
glacis	goffered	gradine	grenache
glacises	goffering	grads	grenadier

GeoSpell French: Spelling Bee Words

grenadine	grivoiseries	guitar	haversack
grenatite	grognard	gyroscope	hectare
gres	gros	gyrovague	hectogram
greses	grosgrain	habile	hectoliter
gridelin	group	habitue	hectometer
griffonage	groupment	hache	helepole
griffonne	grume	hachure	helepoles
grill	guenon	hachures	helepolis
grillade	gueridon	halloysite	helepolises
grillage	gueridons	hangar	helicopter
grimace	guerite	harangued	heliochromy
grimme	guetapens	harass	heliographic
grimoire	guichet	harassed	heliography
grimp	guigne	haricot	heliogravure
gringolee	guignes	harmonichord	heliometer
griot	guignol	harmonium	heliometric
grippe	guignolet	harmotome	hemeralope
grisaille	guillemet	hash	hemicycle
grisard	guillemot	hatchure	hemitropism
grisette	guilloche	hatchures	hemorrhage
grisettish	guillotine	haut	hemorrhoidal
grison	guimbard	hautboist	heraldic
grivet	guimpe	haute	herborize
grivois	guipure	haute-lisse	hermaphrodism
grivoiserie	guisard	hauteur	herniotomy

GeoSpell French: Spelling Bee Words

heroism	houri	ideologue	impressionism
hessonite	humanize	ideology	impromptu
heterosite	humboldtine	idiomography	impromptus
hieroglyph	humid	idocrase	improprieties
hieroglyphics	humidify	idrialite	impropriety
hieroglyphs	hureaulite	igneri	improvise
hippogriff	huron	ignore	impuissant
histology	hydroa	illegal	impure
historiette	hydrogen	illinois	imputable
histotroph	hygiene	imerinite	inamissible
histotrophe	hygrometry	imidogen	inanity
hoc	hypersthene	immeubles	incapacity
hominization	hypnotic	immobilism	incompetence
hominized	hypochondriac	immobilize	inconnu
homotropal	hypocrise	immortelle	incroyable
homotropous	hypogastric	immunist	incunable
hoopla	hypogee	impasse	indecision
hordein	hypothec	impayable	indicolite
horopter	hysterostomatomy	impeditive	indienne
horopteric	ichthyolite	impermeabilization	individualism
hospice	ichthyolitic	impermeabilize	indolence
hotel	iconology	impertinence	indolency
hotelier	ideal	impregnation	indri
houdan	idealogy	impressionable	indris
houppelande	ideologist	impressionableness	indubitable

GeoSpell French: Spelling Bee Words

ineligible	intendant	iodate	jansenism
inept	intermede	iodic	Jansenist
ineri	intern	iodine	japonaiserie
inextirpable	internation	irascibility	japonism
infantine	internationale	iroquois	jardiniere
infaust	interned	Islamic	jargon
inflammable	internment	isochronism	jargoon
inflammableness	interstice	isolation	jasmine
infructescence	interstices	isothere	jaspachate
ingeniosity	intertextuality	isotherm	jaspagate
ingenue	intime	isothermal	jaspe
ingerence	intimidation	iura	jeremejevite
ingerences	intimist	izard	jeremiad
inhumation	intolerance	jabot	jessamine
insectology	intolerant	jacamar	jete
insipid	intrados	jacinthe	jeton
insipidity	intrait	jacobsite	jetton
insolation	intransigeance	jacot	jeu
insouciance	intrigant	jacquerie	jeux
insouciant	intrigante	jadeite	jezekite
inspissation	intrigue	jalap	jocism
installation	introuvable	jalapa	jocist
intangible	intumescence	jalouse	jocko
integrant	invination	jalousie	joinder
intendance	involucre	jalousies	jonglery

GeoSpell French: Spelling Bee Words

jongleur	kilometer	lampion	layette
journalism	kinkajou	lampist	leadhillite
jouvence	kongsbergite	lampistry	lechatelierite
jube	koninckite	lampoon	legionnaire
julienne	kotschubeite	lanarkite	legitim
jumart	kyrielle	lande	legitimism
jumelle	labadism	langouste	legume
jurassic	lacis	langoustine	legumes
jurisprudence	lacroixite	langue	legumin
jus	lactic	lansquenet	lemonade
justaucorps	lactiferous	lapin	leno
justiciable	lactiferousness	lardon	leporide
justicoat	lacune	lardoon	leprosery
juvenile	lagoon	larigot	lerot
kaolin	lai	larmier	levee
karite	laicity	larmoyant	lexicology
keloid	laine	lascive	liaison
keloidal	lais	latanier	liana
kelts	laisse	lateen	liane
kepi	laitance	latrine	lianoid
kermes	lamantin	lavage	liberticidal
kermesite	lamasery	lavaliere	liberticide
kern	lambrequin	lavandin	librettist
khedive	lame	lavaret	liebenerite
kiloliter	lampadite	lawrencite	lienteric

GeoSpell French: Spelling Bee Words

lierne	lipothymic	locule	lucerne
lierre	lipothymy	locules	ludic
ligne	liqueur	locustelle	luge
lignify	liquidity	loge	luminaire
lignite	liroconite	loges	luth
lignitic	lisse	logistics	luthier
ligurite	lisses	loir	lycee
lilac	listel	longe	lyonnaise
lilas	lithoclase	longeron	lyriform
limacel	lithomancy	longitudinal	macabre
limacon	lithophyte	longueur	macaque
limbic	lithotome	lorette	macaroon
liminary	lithotomist	lorgnette	macaroons
limitrophe	litre	lorgnettes	maccaboy
limon	litterateur	lorgnon	macedoine
limonin	livid	loriot	mache
limousin	lividity	lotte	machicotage
limousine	lividness	lotto	machicoulis
limousines	livraison	louche	machicoulises
limpid	livre	loucheux	mackle
lingerie	locality	louis	macle
linon	loche	loupe	macon
lioncel	locomobile	loure	macouba
lipothymia	locomobility	loutre	macquereau
lipothymial	locomotive	lucarne	macquereaux

GeoSpell French: Spelling Bee Words

macrame	maigers	malinger	manifestative
macrocephalic	maigre	malingering	manioc
macrocephalous	maigres	malinois	manioca
macrocosm	maillot	mallardite	mannequin
macrophage	maisonette	malleability	mannite
macrophagic	majuscule	mals	manoir
maculature	maki	maltose	manometer
macule	mal	maltreat	manometric
madame	malacolite	malvoisie	manometrical
madeleine	malacology	mameliere	manometry
mademoiselle	maladroit	mamelon	manque
mademoiselles	malaise	mammiferous	mansard
madrague	malapropos	mamsell	manteau
madrepore	malate	manchineel	manucode
madrigalesque	malaxage	mandeism	maquette
madrilene	malbrouck	mandioc	maquillage
maerl	malchus	mandioca	maquis
magdalenian	malebranchism	mandrin	maquisard
magistrature	malebranchist	manege	marabou
magnesite	maleic	maneuver	marabout
magnetic	malentendu	maneuverer	maraud
magnetize	malgache	manganese	marauding
magot	malgre	mangue	marc
mahoe	malic	manicure	marcot
maiger	maline	manifestant	marcottage

GeoSpell French: Spelling Bee Words

marengo	marteline	mattamore	melanose
margarin	martenot	matte	melaphyre
margarine	martiniquais	mattoir	melee
margay	marver	mauve	melegueta
marguerite	mascaron	mauvette	melezitose
marianna	mascot	mayonnaise	melilite
marianne	masculinity	mazagran	melinite
marigraph	massage	meagre	melomane
maringouin	masse	meconin	melongene
marionette	massecuite	medaillon	memoir
marionettes	masseur	medalist	menage
marist	masseuse	medallion	menagerie
marli	massif	medical	menhir
marmit	massifs	medicamentous	menilite
marmite	mastigoneme	medication	menopause
marmot	matamoro	medin	menton
marocain	matelasse	mediocracy	menu
maroquin	matelot	medoc	mephitic
marotte	matelote	megass	mephitical
marouflage	materiel	mehari	mercantile
marquessate	maternity	meharist	mercantilism
marquise	mathurin	meionite	meridienne
marron	matinal	melange	meringue
marseillais	matinee	melangeur	merlon
martele	matlow	melanian	merlot

GeoSpell French: Spelling Bee Words

merovingian	metrician	milieux	mistigris
mesalliance	metro	militarism	mistral
mesalliances	metrology	militarize	mitoclasic
mesange	metropole	millefleur	mitraille
mesclun	metropoly	millefleurs	mitrailleuse
mesdames	metros	millegrain	mittle
mesdemoiselles	meubles	milliard	mobiliary
mesenteric	meuniere	millieme	mobilize
meshrabiyeh	meursault	milligram	modality
mesoseme	mezzanine	milliliter	moderantism
messaline	miasmatic	millionaire	moderantist
messeigneurs	miaul	milord	moderne
mesvinian	miauled	minaret	modiste
metagnomy	microfiche	minauderie	mofette
metayage	micrometer	minauderies	moire
metayer	midinette	minaudiere	molasse
meteorism	mignon	minionette	molasses
meteorology	mignonette	ministrable	molecule
methylene	mignonne	minuscule	molecules
metier	migraine	mirabelle	mollusk
metif	migration	mirage	molybdomenite
metifs	migrational	mirepoix	monadology
metis	milady	mirliton	monarchism
metisse	milanaise	misere	monastic
metisses	milieu	mistelle	mondaine

GeoSpell French: Spelling Bee Words

mondial	monzonite	motif	municipality
monegasque	monzonitic	motocross	muriate
monocarp	moquette	mots	musar
monocle	moraine	moucharaby	muscade
monocoque	morale	mouchoir	muscadet
monodactyle	morceau	moue	muscadin
monogamy	morceaus	mouflon	muscardine
monolith	morceaux	mouille	muscat
monolithic	morcellation	mouillure	musculature
monologue	morcellement	moulage	museography
monophysism	mordore	moulin	musette
monseigneur	morel	mousquetaire	musicale
montage	morelles	mousse	musketry
montagnais	moresque	mousseline	muslin
montagnaises	morgue	Mousterian	mutage
montagnard	morillon	mozabite	mutism
montagnards	morin	mozarabic	myology
montaignesque	morinite	mucosity	myope
montebrasite	morne	muet	myriameter
monticle	morpheme	mugho	myriameters
monticule	morphemic	muguet	mysticity
montmartrite	morphine	mulattress	mystification
montrachet	morphological	multiform	mystificator
montre	mortier	multiple	mystify
monture	mot	multipliable	mystique

GeoSpell French: Spelling Bee Words

mythologize	narratologist	niche	nonchalance
mythologizer	narratology	nickeline	nonchalant
mythology	natality	nicoise	nonillion
nabi	natchez	nicotine	nontronite
nacarat	natromontebrasite	nigerois	nonuple
nacelle	natron	nihilist	nordic
nacre	natte	nihility	normative
nacrite	navarin	nitrate	nougat
nadiral	nazard	nitriary	nouveau
nadorite	nebulosity	nitric	nouvelle
nagor	necessitous	nitrification	novitiate
naiad	nee	nitrify	nowy
naiades	nef	nitrogen	noyade
naiads	negligee	niveau	nuance
naissance	negress	noachite	nubile
naive	negritude	noctambule	nubility
naivete	neocomian	noctilucine	nuciform
nanger	neologism	nocturne	nucule
nanism	neology	nodosity	nudiped
nanization	nepotism	noel	nudity
nappe	nervure	noir	nul
narceine	neufchatel	noirs	numerator
narcotine	neumatic	noisette	numismatics
narcotism	neume	noisettes	nummiform
narratological	neve	nomancy	nummular

GeoSpell French: Spelling Bee Words

nuptiality	octuor	oligistical	opting
nymphaeum	oculist	oliphant	option
nymphal	odalisque	olivette	opts
oblat	odometer	ombre	opuscule
obligement	odontalgic	omelet	orangeade
obole	odontolite	omnibus	orangerie
obscenity	odontology	ondine	orangery
obscurant	oeillade	ondograph	orcein
obscurantism	oeillades	ondule	orchesography
obscurement	oeuvre	onomancy	orchestrate
obsede	oeuvres	onomatology	orchestration
observable	officiality	onomatopoeic	orchestrelle
observant	ogival	opacity	ordonnance
obtention	ogive	operon	oreide
obus	ogre	ophicleide	orfevrerie
obuses	ogress	ophicleidean	organdy
occitan	oka	ophiolite	organoleptic
oceanian	oke	ophiolitic	organzine
oceanic	okoume	opinant	orgeat
ocelot	oleate	opisthogastric	orgue
ochlocrat	oleiculture	opportunist	orguinette
octahedrite	olein	opt	orientate
octillion	oleine	optician	originality
octobass	oligist	optimism	orillon
octroi	oligistic	optimist	oriole

GeoSpell French: Spelling Bee Words

orlean	ottoman	paillasse	palmierite
orleanist	ottrelite	paillasson	palmitin
ormer	ouabaio	paillette	palpitant
ormolu	oubliette	paillon	pampre
oroide	outre	paintress	panachage
orpheon	outreness	pairle	panache
orpheonist	ouvert	pajonism	panached
orpheons	oviscapt	paladin	panachure
orphist	ovoid	palafitte	panary
orseille	ovoidal	palafitti	panda
orselle	oxalate	palais	pandiculation
orthodromy	oxidable	palaises	pandour
orthopedic	oxidant	palatal	panetiere
orthopedist	oxidation	palatally	panne
orthopter	oxide	paleontography	pantagruelism
orthosite	oxygen	paleontology	pantheism
ortolan	oxygenate	paletot	pantine
orvietan	oxygenation	palette	pantometer
oryzivorous	oxytone	palfrenier	pantoum
oscule	pachyderm	palingenesy	paon
osselet	pacifism	palisade	papalist
ostensible	pacifist	palisades	papelonne
otolith	pagne	palliative	papeterie
otolithic	pagodite	pallisades	papeteries
ottawa	paillard	palmette	papillary

GeoSpell French: Spelling Bee Words

papillon	parmone	passerelle	paysanne
papillote	parodist	pastiche	pearlite
papoosh	parole	pasticheur	pearlitic
papyrin	paroli	pastille	pebrine
papyrine	paroxysm	pastis	pebrinous
paquebot	parquet	pataphysics	pectic
parachute	parquetage	patas	pectin
parachutic	parquetry	pate	pectoriloquy
parade	parsonsite	pathologic	pedalier
parades	parterre	pathological	pedantocracy
parados	parti	patine	pedantry
paralyze	partis	patisserie	pedicule
paraphrastic	partism	patissier	pedicure
paraphrastical	parure	patois	pediform
parasol	parvenu	patrol	pedometer
paravent	parvenue	patronne	pegmatite
paregoric	paspies	patroon	peignoir
parfait	paspy	paturon	pekin
parisian	passacaille	paupiette	pelage
parisianism	passade	pave	pelerine
parisienne	passe	pavillon	pelisse
parison	passecaille	pavisade	peloton
parme	passementerie	paysage	penchant
parmentier	passepied	paysagist	penche
parmentiere	passepieds	paysagiste	pendeloque

GeoSpell French: Spelling Bee Words

pendentive	perioplic	pervenche	pharyngoscope
pendular	peripety	pervertible	phene
pendule	perisperm	pesade	phenocryst
pendulette	perispermal	pessimism	phenocrystic
penetrability	peristyle	pessimist	phialide
penial	perle	petardier	philamot
pensionnat	perleche	petillant	philatelist
pentlandite	perlite	petite	philately
peoria	perloir	petitgrain	philharmonic
percaline	permissive	petrification	philippism
percalines	perrinist	petrissage	philippist
percheron	perron	petroglyph	philippistic
perfectibility	perruche	petroglyphs	philology
perfectible	perscrutation	petulance	philosophe
peridot	persienne	phalange	philosophism
peridote	persiflage	phalangette	phlegmonous
peridotic	persifleur	phalansterian	phloretin
peridotite	persillade	phalanstery	phoneme
peridotitic	personify	phalarope	phonolite
perigone	personnel	phallocracy	phonometry
perijove	perspirable	phallocrat	phosphate
perimeter	perspiration	phallocratic	phosphite
periodic	perspire	phanerogam	phosphor
periodicity	peruginesque	pharaonic	phosphoric
periople	peruker	phare	photogravure

GeoSpell French: Spelling Bee Words

physiocracy	pierrotage	piste	platoon
physiocrat	piety	piston	plats
physionotrace	pignon	pistou	pleasantry
physique	pignorative	pithiviers	plebe
piaffe	pike	piton	plectre
pian	pilotage	pitot	pleiad
pianist	pinard	pivot	pleinairism
pianiste	pinche	plafond	pleinairisme
piaster	pineal	plage	pleinairist
pic	pinot	plaidoyer	pleinairiste
picaillon	piolet	plainchant	pleonaste
picard	pioupiou	plancheite	pleuric
picarel	pipette	planchette	plie
picayune	pipistrelle	planimeter	plies
piccadilly	pique	planimetry	plisse
pickadil	piqued	plantigrade	plombage
pickadilly	piquette	plaque	plumetis
picot	piqueur	plaquette	plurilocular
picotite	pirogue	plastique	pluviometer
picqueter	piroque	plat	pneumatique
picrite	pirouette	platband	pochade
pics	pise	plateau	poche
picucule	pissaladiere	platitude	pochette
pierrette	pissoir	platonician	pochoir
pierrot	pistache	platonize	poil

GeoSpell French: Spelling Bee Words

poilu	pompier	postiche	precieux
pointe	pompon	postulant	precipitant
pointillage	ponceau	posture	precipitous
pointille	pontiff	potager	precis
pointillism	pontil	potiche	predilection
poise	ponton	potichomania	predominance
poivrade	pontonier	potpourri	prefectoral
polacre	pontoon	poudrette	preferable
polarization	poontang	poudreuse	preference
polarize	popeline	pouf	prehensile
polatouche	poplin	poularde	prehensility
polemic	populin	poule	prejudgment
polignac	pornograph	poulette	prelature
polissoir	portail	pourboire	prele
politesse	portefeuille	pourparler	preliminary
politique	portiere	poussette	premiere
polonaise	portugais	poussin	preparateur
polypheme	porty	prairial	prepose
polytheism	poseur	prairie	prepotence
pomarine	poseuse	praiss	presbytere
pomerol	positivism	praline	presentiment
pommard	posology	prase	prestant
pomme	possibilism	pratique	prestidigitation
pommee	possibilist	precaution	prestidigitator
pommel	postface	precieuse	prestidigitatory

GeoSpell French: Spelling Bee Words

prestige	progressism	provenance	pulmonic
presumable	progressist	provencale	punitive
pretentious	prohibitive	province	puntil
preux	projet	provisory	pupillary
prevalence	proletariat	provocateur	puree
prevenance	proliferation	proxenet	purgery
priapism	prolific	proxenete	purism
priapismic	prolonge	prude	purist
primatial	promenade	prudery	putrescibility
primeur	prominence	prunelle	putrescible
printanier	promiscuity	prussiate	putty
prismatic	proneur	psammite	puy
prix	propagandism	psammitic	pycnite
probabiliorism	prophylaxy	psephite	pyrgocephalic
probabiliorist	propolize	psephitic	pyrgocephaly
probabilism	proposant	pseudoboleite	pyric
probabilist	prosaism	pseudonym	pyroligneous
proboscide	prosateur	psychism	pyrolignite
procacity	protege	psychologue	pyrolignous
procedure	protegee	publicist	pyroxene
prodrome	proteiform	publicity	pyrrhonism
professorate	protein	puce	pythonoid
profiterole	protestantism	pudic	quadrillage
profonde	prototype	puericulture	quadrille
progeniture	proustite	puerile	quadrillion

GeoSpell French: Spelling Bee Words

quai	raffinate	rarefaction	recercelee
quais	raffinose	rascasse	rechauffe
quartzose	rafraichissoir	rascette	recherche
quatorze	ragout	ratafia	recidivist
quatrain	raillery	rataplan	recit
quatuor	railleur	ratatouille	recitatif
quebecois	rais	ratine	reclame
quenelle	raisine	ration	recollection
questeur	rale	ravage	reconnaissance
questionnaire	rallies	ravigote	reconnoiter
quete	rally	ravine	recoup
quiche	ramage	ravison	recruit
quillon	ramekin	rayonism	redaction
quinte	ramification	rayonnant	redan
quinton	ramism	razee	redemptorist
quintons	ramist	razzia	redhibition
quinzaine	ramoneur	reactionary	redingote
rab	ranche	readjourn	redoppe
rabbin	rapide	realization	redoubt
racemic	rappee	realize	redowa
rachidian	rappel	realized	refait
raclette	rapport	rebarbative	reflet
raconteur	rapportage	reblochon	refugee
raconteuse	rapporteur	reboise	refusion
rafale	rapprochement	reboisement	regale

GeoSpell French: Spelling Bee Words

regaled	rentier	respirable	rever
regalian	renverse	ressaulted	reverie
regence	renversement	restaur	reveries
regie	renvoi	restaurant	revers
regime	repartee	restaurateur	reversi
regisseur	repechage	restauration	reversis
reglementary	repertoire	restauratrice	revet
regularity	repetiteur	resume	revete
rejoindure	repoussage	retable	revetement
releve	repousse	reticence	revetment
reliquary	representant	reticule	revision
remanie	reprimand	retinite	revivified
remarkable	republic	retirade	revivify
remarque	requin	retouch	revue
remiped	reseau	retrace	revuist
remontant	reseaus	retree	rexist
remoulade	reseaux	retro	rhapsode
renaissance	resentment	retroactive	rhodeswood
renal	reservoir	retroussage	rhum
renardite	reservoirs	retrousse	rhyparographic
rendition	resignatary	revanche	richellite
rendu	resiliate	revanchism	ricochet
renifleur	resinification	reveillon	rideau
renitent	resinify	revenant	rideaus
rente	resource	revendication	ridicule

GeoSpell French: Spelling Bee Words

rigadoon	rompu	roussette	sagaie
rigadoons	roncet	routine	sagenite
rigaudons	rondache	roux	sagoin
rigorism	ronde	royale	sahel
riguadon	rongeur	ruade	sahelian
rilletts	ronier	rubasse	saic
rinceau	roquelaure	ruche	sainfoin
rinceaux	roquette	rudenture	saintfoin
riposte	rorqual	ruse	sajou
risk	rosace	rustre	saki
risque	rose	sabayon	salangane
rissole	rosette	sabbat	salariat
riverain	rosieresite	saber	saleb
riviere	rotisserie	sabir	saleeite
robespierrist	roucou	sabot	salep
rocaille	roue	sabotage	salicin
rocambole	rouge	saboteur	salify
rococo	rougeot	sabotier	salinelle
rocou	rouget	sabotiers	salle
rogatory	rouille	sabretache	salmagundi
rognon	roulade	sabreur	salmi
role	rouleau	sac	salon
romaine	rouleaux	saccade	salons
romantic	roulette	sachet	saloon
romantism	rouman	sadic	salse

GeoSpell French: Spelling Bee Words

salsify	sarcocarp	sauvegarde	secateur
salteaux	sarcode	savant	secateurs
saltimbanco	sard	savarin	seconde
salvage	sardinier	savate	secretage
samarskite	sardiniers	savonnerie	secretaire
samiresite	sards	savoy	secretion
sancerre	sarrazin	Savoyard	secularization
sanfoin	satinay	saxe	secularize
sangfroid	satine	saxophone	sedative
sangsue	satirize	saynete	seiche
sanitary	satrapy	scapolite	seigneurial
sansculotte	satyric	scaramouch	seigneury
sansculotterie	saucier	schapska	semainier
sansculottism	saucisson	schist	semanteme
santal	saulteur	scissel	semantics
santon	saurel	scissile	semble
sapajou	saussurite	scission	semeed
saponification	saussuritic	scotch	semis
saponify	saute	sculpt	semite
saponin	sauterelle	scutch	semnopitheque
sappare	sauterne	scytodepsic	semy
saraband	sauternes	seance	senegalese
sarbacane	sauteur	seau	senonian
sarbican	sautille	seaux	sensibilize
sarcasm	sautoir	sec	sentiment

GeoSpell French: Spelling Bee Words

septennate	seybertite	sirvents	solitaire
septieme	seychellois	sixain	solleret
septier	shako	sixte	solmization
septillion	sharpite	sklodowskite	somber
septleva	shivaree	slovincian	sommelier
sequin	siberite	smaltite	somnial
serac	siffleur	smaragdite	sondage
serandite	sigillography	sobriquet	sondages
sercial	signifie	societaire	sonde
serein	silhouette	sociocracy	sortie
serenade	silique	sociology	sosie
serf	silviculture	socle	sotie
sericiculture	simar	soffit	sou
serin	similar	soffite	souari
serinette	simplify	soigne	soubise
serosity	simplism	soiree	soubresaut
serpentin	sinaite	solanin	soubrette
serpierite	singerie	solanine	soubriquet
serpolet	singleton	soleil	souffle
serrefine	sinologue	solenoid	souffleed
serval	sioux	solfege	soufriere
serviette	siphon	solidarity	soukous
servomotor	siroc	solidarize	souletin
sesban	sirop	solidary	soup
sextillion	sirventes	soliste	soupcon

GeoSpell French: Spelling Bee Words

souple	spontoon	stylet	surjection
sourdine	sporule	styracin	surmullet
souriquois	squame	suberate	surrealism
sous	statuette	suberin	surtout
soutache	staurolite	suberone	surveillance
soutane	staurolitic	succinic	surveillant
souteneur	staurotide	succinite	survivance
soutenu	stearic	succulence	suzerain
souterrain	stearin	succumb	suzerainty
souvenir	stearine	succursal	svelte
souverain	stephanian	sucrier	sylphid
spadille	stere	suint	sylvanite
sparterie	stereid	suite	sylvite
specter	stereobate	suivez	symbiot
spessartine	stereotomy	sulpician	symbiote
spessartite	stereotype	sultanate	syndactyl
spet	steres	sultane	syndactylic
sphene	stethoscope	Sumerian	syndactylous
spilite	stilbite	superposition	syndic
spilitic	strass	sur	syndical
spinulous	stratosphere	surbased	syndicalism
spirituel	stridulation	surette	syndicalist
splenification	strie	surface	syntax
splenization	strophoid	suricat	syphilization
sponton	strychnine	suricate	syphilize

GeoSpell French: Spelling Bee Words

syrah	tamanoir	tartine	tepal
syringin	tamarin	Tartuffery	terebene
tabby	tambour	tastevin	terebenthene
tableau	tamis	tatbeb	terfez
tableaus	tamises	taupe	terrain
tableaux	tampon	tautochrone	terrasse
taboret	tanghin	taximeter	terrier
tacheometer	tannate	taxonomy	terrine
tachism	tannic	tayacian	terrorism
tachist	tannin	tchaviche	terrorist
tachygraph	tantieme	technique	tete
tachymetry	tanystome	teil	thalassic
tacit	tapeinocephalism	telegraph	thalenite
taciturn	tapeinocephaly	telegraphist	thaumaturg
tact	tapissier	templet	thaumaturge
tactician	tapotement	temps	theatral
tactile	tardigrade	tenable	thelemite
tafia	tardive	tenaillon	thenardite
taille	tarente	tenaillons	theorician
tailleur	tarlatan	tendresse	theosoph
talapoin	tarleton	tendu	thermidor
talisman	tarsier	tenrec	thermidorean
talmouse	tartana	tensive	thermometer
talmouses	tartane	tenson	thonnier
talus	tartarin	tenue	thoracic

GeoSpell French: Spelling Bee Words

thoreaulite	tonne	tourniquet	travesty
tibourbou	tonneau	tournure	treillage
tierce	tontine	tourte	tremblement
tierced	topazolite	trachyandesite	tremie
tierceron	topinambour	trachyte	tremolite
tige	torchere	trachytic	tremolitic
tigress	torchon	trachytoid	trephine
tilleul	tordion	traineau	triage
timariot	tordions	traineaux	tribade
timbale	tore	traiteur	tribadic
timoneer	torque	trajet	triblet
tinamou	torrent	tram	tribometer
tintamarre	torsade	tranche	tricolor
tiqueur	tortille	tranchet	tricot
tirade	tortillon	transgress	tricotine
tirasse	torture	transhumance	trictrac
tisane	toucan	transhumant	tricycle
titer	touche	transhumantes	trigone
toile	toupet	transvase	trillion
toilette	tourelle	transversale	trimester
tole	tourlourou	trapeze	trimestrial
tolerant	tournasin	trappist	tringle
tombe	tournedos	travail	trio
Tomme	tournette	travails	triolet
tonlet	tourneur	travaux	tripery

GeoSpell French: Spelling Bee Words

triphane	tudesque	urceiform	vaudeville
tripoli	tuillette	urethan	vedette
troat	tukuler	urethane	vehicle
trocar	Tukulor	urticant	velo
trochee	tulle	utilization	velociman
troke	turbine	utilize	velocipede
troker	turonian	vaccination	velodrome
trompil	tutoyer	vacherin	velour
troostitic	tutu	vacillation	velours
trophic	tuyere	vacuole	veloute
trotteur	tweel	vacuome	venality
trottoir	tylose	vagabondage	vendeuse
troubadour	typic	valise	vendue
troupe	tyrannicide	valois	venise
trousseau	tyrolienne	valse	ventral
trousseaux	tzigane	vampire	ventripotent
trouvaille	ukase	vandalism	venturine
trouve	ukaz	vandenbrandeite	verbiage
trouvere	unanimism	vandenbrandite	verdin
trumeau	unau	vanille	verglas
trumeaux	unique	vanillery	verglases
trunnion	univoltine	vanillon	verite
trunnioned	uran	varec	vernissage
tubercule	urate	varsovienne	veronique
tubulure	urbanism	vase	versatile

GeoSpell French: Spelling Bee Words

versatility	vigoureux	vivres	voyeur
versicule	villiaumite	vocalise	vraic
verst	vinage	vocalises	vrille
verve	vinaigrette	voeu	wehrlite
verveine	vinaigrettes	voeux	wernerite
vervelle	vinasse	voila	wistit
vervet	vinification	voile	wurtzite
vesical	violine	voilier	wurtzitic
vesperale	virement	voiture	xanthic
vespetro	virgule	voiturette	xanthophyll
vestibule	visa	vol	xenotime
vestige	vis-a-vis	volborthite	xylindein
vetiver	viscin	volcanic	xylography
vetivert	vise	volcanicity	yperite
veuve	viseite	vole	zaire
veuves	visitandine	volet	zebu
viability	visite	volition	zero
viable	vison	volplane	zest
vibratile	vite	volt	zigzag
vibratility	vitrailed	voltigeur	ziryen
vicereine	vitraillist	vomition	zoril
vichyssoise	vitrify	Vosgian	zorilla
vide	vitrine	vouge	zorille
vielle	vivandiere	voussoir	zorillo
vignette	viveur	vouvray	zouave

GeoSpell French: Spelling Bee Words

Words from Medieval French:

abdomen	affability	amass	archduke
abeyance	affable	ambuscade	architecture
abolition	affianced	amortizement	architrave
absterge	affiant	ampliation	aristocracy
abstersive	affine	anagram	arithmetician
abstraction	affirmance	anatomize	armet
absurd	affirmation	anfractuosity	armillary
abusive	affreight	angelot	armoire
accent	agate	angular	aromatize
acceptance	aggrandizement	annuity	arpen
accession	agile	annular	arpent
accost	agist	annulet	arterial
accouplement	agistment	antique	artifice
accoutrement	agitation	aphorism	artisan
acerbity	agog	apology	asperge
acidify	aidance	apostatize	assailant
aconite	aider	apostil	assart
acrimony	alamort	appellee	assassinate
acrostic	alexandrine	appendance	assegai
activity	allotment	appetitive	ataraxia
acuity	alloy	applaud	ataraxy
adhere	almuce	apportion	atheism
adoration	aludel	appose	atrocity
adornment	aluminous	arable	attornment

GeoSpell French: Spelling Bee Words

audition	beatify	bricole	canonist
augmentative	beauseant	brulyie	canton
avenue	bedeguar	buccan	caparison
avowant	beguine	buffoon	capitulation
axunge	benzoin	bugloss	capture
bailment	bernicle	bulbous	capuchin
baize	bevel	burgonet	capuchine
baladine	bezoar	burse	caravel
bandage	biggin	cabinet	carcass
bandoleer	bigot	cabochon	carnage
bandolier	bilious	cachet	carob
bandy	bistort	calamity	caroche
bannerol	bombardier	calender	carouse
banquet	bombasine	caliber	carrefour
barbery	bombazine	caliginous	cartel
bardash	botonee	callet	cartilaginous
barde	botonny	callosity	caruncle
barding	bouget	callous	casemate
barretter	bourgeois	calumniator	cassock
barricade	brankursine	calumny	catacomb
basil	branle	camaieu	catacombs
bastide	bravado	camaieux	cataplasm
bastion	bravery	cannon	catapult
battalion	brawl	cannonade	catarrh
battery	bretesse	cannoneer	catarrhal

GeoSpell French: Spelling Bee Words

catarrhally	chirograph	comedian	consign
cauter	chiromancy	comestible	consistence
cauterize	chopine	commendable	contemner
cavalcade	cicatrization	commensurability	contend
cavalier	cicatrize	commensurable	contingency
cavity	circulation	commentation	continuity
cecity	citadel	commerce	contravallation
cent	cite	commiseration	contravene
cents	clandestine	compartment	contrist
cephalic	clavel	compatible	contumelious
cesser	cleromancy	competence	contuse
cestui	clinquant	competitor	convalescence
chace	coalition	compony	convex
chammy	cochineal	comport	convexity
chamois	codicil	comportment	copiosity
chamoix	cogitative	concert	coppice
champertor	coherence	concussion	cordage
champignon	coherent	condolence	cordon
chapeau	cohort	condolences	cornice
chapeaux	colleague	conference	coronet
chard	collegial	conferrence	corpulence
chatelain	collet	congelative	corridor
chevaline	coloss	congratulations	corrival
chewet	combatant	conjugal	corroboration
chirognomy	combustible	connex	corsair

GeoSpell French: Spelling Bee Words

corselet	cynic	depilation	dissuade
coruscation	cynosure	descendance	dissuasion
cosmolabe	daker	desinence	docility
cotehardie	damageable	despot	domain
cotise	debauch	dessert	domicil
cottier	debel	detainer	domicile
couplet	debility	determinator	dominant
courante	decadence	detersive	dormition
courier	decent	deuce	dowager
courtesan	decision	devest	druggery
coutel	declamation	devow	ducal
crampon	declension	dexterity	ductile
crampoon	decrepitude	dialectician	dullard
crenel	defray	difficile	eaglet
crenele	deific	difformity	eclogue
crenelle	delinquent	dignify	ecu
cribble	demicannon	digue	ecus
criminous	demilance	diopter	efface
crinet	demission	dioptre	effigy
croche	demit	direption	elegance
croze	democracy	discernment	eloge
crudity	demolish	disputable	eloges
crural	demurrer	dissonance	embark
cubeb	denticule	dissonancy	embassy
curative	dentifrice	dissonant	empale

GeoSpell French: Spelling Bee Words

enceinte	espringal	fecal	futile
enforcement	essay	fermail	gabardine
englut	estoile	filament	gaberdine
engorge	estoppel	fisc	gabion
engrave	estrepe	fitchee	gager
enormity	eternize	flamant	galactite
enrage	evade	flancard	galleass
ensorcell	excision	flatulent	gallery
entrain	excitative	fluviatile	galliard
entrap	exigence	fluxion	gallimaufry
epact	extenuation	formativeness	gallop
epilepsy	fabulist	formulary	garniture
equidistant	facetious	fourrier	garrulity
equipage	facile	fouter	gauze
equipped	faction	foutra	gean
equipt	factious	friable	gendarmerie
equitation	factory	friableness	genteel
equivalence	faerie	fricassee	gigot
equivalency	fallacious	friction	glanders
erminites	falsification	frigate	gleek
erminois	farthingale	frippery	gluten
erosion	fash	frugal	glutenous
escrow	fasherie	fruitage	glutinous
escuage	fatality	fulmination	goff
esplees	fatuity	furor	gool

GeoSpell French: Spelling Bee Words

gormand	habitant	hostility	incised
gourmand	hackbut	hotch	incitation
grandiloquence	hackbuteer	huguenot	incite
grapple	hackbutter	huguenotic	incommode
gratify	hagbut	huitain	incompetent
gratuity	halberdier	humetty	incongruity
gravity	harquebus	humoral	indication
greffier	harquebusier	hutchet	inelegant
grenade	hautbois	icteric	inexpugnable
grogram	hazardous	idiom	infantry
grot	heaume	idiotism	infest
grotesque	helmet	ignominious	infidel
guaranty	hemorrhoid	ignominy	infidelity
guardant	hennin	impale	infractor
guidon	herborist	impart	ingenious
guttee	hereditable	impetuosity	inhuman
guttural	heredity	impiety	inimitable
gutturalism	heteroclite	improbation	inquisitor
gutturality	hippodrome	impudicity	insipient
gutty	histrion	impuissance	intellective
gymnast	horde	impulsive	intensive
gyration	horoscope	impunity	intercalation
gyromancy	horrific	inaccessible	interpel
gyron	hostile	incarnadine	interpose
habiliment	hostilities	incise	interreign

GeoSpell French: Spelling Bee Words

intestinal	lagend	lohoch	mathematician
intitule	lament	looch	median
intrinsic	lampas	lottery	mediocre
introit	lancer	lowy	metaphor
inveigle	landgraviate	lubricity	meteorological
irascible	langued	lunette	metrify
irritant	languid	luster	meuse
isabel	languorous	magazine	military
isabella	lassitude	maladive	minion
islet	legerity	malevolence	ministress
italianism	legist	maltolte	minot
iterative	lenitive	malversation	miraculous
ivray	lethargic	mandate	mirific
jactance	liard	mandible	mise
jactancy	licit	mandilion	misfeasance
javelin	lien	maniable	mobile
judicature	lientery	mantel	mobility
judicious	lieu	marquetry	monachism
jurist	ligation	martel	monarchical
laceration	linnet	martin	monomachy
lachrymal	lionet	martingale	monsieur
lackey	liquefy	martlet	monstrance
laconism	lobe	masque	mordant
ladrone	lodgment	masquerade	morion
lagan	logan	massacre	morpion

GeoSpell French: Spelling Bee Words

mournival	nebule	obtest	pacification
moustache	nebuly	occipital	packet
muleteer	negatory	octroy	palinody
multiplicity	neutral	ode	palliation
mummer	neutrality	offensible	palped
mummery	nicotian	oleaginous	pansy
mundanity	nocive	olympiad	pantalone
mundify	nocturnal	omoplate	pantaloon
munificence	nombril	operative	papable
muniment	nonpareil	operativeness	papism
munition	notoriety	opine	paragon
muscle	null	opiniative	parallax
musketoon	nullity	oppression	paralogism
mutineer	numerosity	optative	paraph
myrabolam	nuque	optatively	parietal
myrabolan	nyctalope	optic	parlance
myrobalam	nymphet	orc	parley
myrobalan	obelisk	orcanette	parmesan
mysterious	obfusque	orgy	parol
naif	objurgation	orifice	particule
naissant	oblectation	orle	partisan
narrative	obscene	ornature	pasquin
naturality	obscurity	ors	pasquinade
navet	observator	orthodox	passament
navette	obtemper	owelty	passant

GeoSpell French: Spelling Bee Words

passement	pernicious	pistole	potage
pastel	persistence	placation	potencee
pastern	persuasible	plancier	pottery
pasturage	persuasive	planish	poulaine
paternity	persuasively	plastron	precipice
pathetic	pertinacity	platen	precise
patonce	pertinency	plumassier	predicant
pattee	peruke	plumet	predicator
paty	petard	poetize	predominant
pavane	petrarchize	poetizer	prefixion
pean	petrify	poignard	prejacent
peccable	petrol	poitrel	prejudge
pedant	petrous	poltroon	prelude
pedestal	phenicopter	poltroonery	premonition
pensionary	philippic	polygamy	prescriptible
pensionnaire	philologer	polyp	presidence
peopling	philologue	pomade	pretendant
peregrination	philter	pommelly	probability
peregrinity	phlebotomize	poniard	probity
perfume	pilaster	populace	procureur
periapt	pilot	porcelain	prophetic
perigee	pincette	portmanteau	provencal
periphery	pinnace	possessive	proximity
periphrase	pioneer	postilion	pudicity
perjure	piquant	postpose	puerility

GeoSpell French: Spelling Bee Words

pumpet	recusation	rodomontade	scene
punaise	refrigerant	rodomontado	sciatic
punese	reginal	rondeau	scimitar
puny	reminiscence	rondeaux	scrupulosity
quatorzain	reminiscences	rondelet	scurrile
quietude	remissible	roturier	scurrility
quinquereme	remonstrance	ruffian	secours
quintuple	rencontre	rusticity	sectator
rabat	rencounter	sackbut	sedentary
racket	rendezvous	safflower	sediment
ramify	renouncement	sagacity	seduction
rampart	repulsion	salacity	seigneur
rampire	requisition	salic	seme
rapacity	rescription	salique	sentinel
rapier	resile	salivation	serail
rasure	retardance	sanctimony	serenity
ratiocination	retirement	sanguification	serous
ravelin	revie	sarcelly	serry
rayon	rhomb	sashoon	sestine
rebatement	rhomboid	satellite	setier
rebec	rhythm	satiety	severe
rebuff	riant	satire	severity
recision	rigid	scandalous	sew
recrement	rival	scarab	shallop
rectory	roan	scarabee	sideral

GeoSpell French: Spelling Bee Words

sincere	suborn	tartan	transpirable
sincerity	subornation	tass	tret
sinople	sue	tasse	triplication
situation	sullage	tenaille	trochaic
skiff	sullied	tenne	trouveur
smalt	sully	terrace	trover
society	sultan	terreplein	tuberosity
solidity	summar	teston	tuff
somersault	sumptuosity	testoon	tumefaction
sorbet	sumptuous	theologian	tumefy
sordine	superbity	tier	turban
souse	superiority	tiers	turpitude
sparge	suppliantly	timbre	tyrannize
spermatic	surge	timocracy	unison
spheric	suture	tocsin	urbanity
spinach	symbolize	toise	urgence
spinney	tablature	toque	ustion
squad	taborin	torse	utile
squash	tainture	torteaux	vacance
stade	talc	tourbillion	valet
stance	tambourine	tragacanth	validity
stradiot	tamper	tragedienne	valuation
stupefy	tarot	tragicomedy	varvel
stupefying	tarots	trait	vaudois
suave	tarragon	transpierce	vehemence

GeoSpell French: Spelling Bee Words

velocity	vesication	viols	vogue
vendor	vesicatory	viper	volant
veneur	vesicle	virile	volley
venue	viceroy	vituperous	voluble
verbosity	vicinity	vivandier	vomitive
verdant	vicissitude	vive	voracity
verdet	vidame	vively	voucher
verditer	vigilance	vivify	walloon
veritable	viol	vocable	zibeline
vervel	violon	vocabulary	

GeoSpell French: Spelling Bee Words

Words from American French:

bamboche	chicot	file	pape
cabouca	choupique	gourde	prairillon
cafe brulot	christophine	gumbo	rigolet
calumet	combite	lagniappe	
chenier	coumbite	palmiste	

Words from Anglo-French:

alienor	essoiner	onde	replevisable
amenable	estray	ondy	sokemanry
amenance	estrepement	orb	tolt
conusable	feme	oust	tourn
darrein	femme	paramount	tron
defeasible	gainor	paravail	tronage
deforciant	galilee	parcenary	trone
demisang	gist	pavage	venter
deodand	liable	pernancy	verderer
disseisee	mesnality	personalty	vicontiel
dittander	mesnalty	prisal	vill
doitkin	mesne	puisne	waiver
dowable	misfeasor	pursive	
embraceor	moline	puture	
essoinee	nieve	rebutter	

GeoSpell French: Spelling Bee Words

Words from Canadian-French:

aboideau	caplin	dore	shanty
aboideaux	capling	epinette	siscowet
aboiteau	carcajou	frazil	toboggan
aboiteaux	caribou	gaspereau	togue
babiche	chantecler	habitan	travois
barbooth	chantier	joual	travoise
barbotte	chantiers	lacrosse	travoy
barbudi	cheyenne	ouananiche	tuladi
bateau	cisco	outarde	tullibee
bateaux	coteau	parfleche	tuque
bois blanc	coteaux	pekan	voyageur
brule	coulie	pembina	watap
brulee	coureur	pimbina	
bunkum	crappie	plew	
capelin	croppie	sagamite	

GeoSpell French: Spelling Bee Words

Words 'modified' or 'probably' from French:

acetate	anthraquinone	calot	coulier
acetic	apace	calycle	courant
acinarious	apivorous	cappo	coxal
actinocrinite	aquafortist	caraibe	coze
actinomere	archivist	carburant	cremorne
adipocere	areometer	carolytic	cromona
adipocerous	armament	carvene	cromorna
aerometer	arviculture	casein	crusie
affranchise	ascophore	catoptromancy	cryptonym
affreightment	ascospore	centimo	cryptophyte
agronomy	atavic	ceromancy	cuneiform
alienable	atonic	chamotte	cutch
alizarin	aurous	chantey	cylindricity
alizarine	autofrettage	charabanc	daiker
alod	axillary	chemism	darning
alphitomorphous	badenite	chinesery	declarator
alveolar	bonapartism	chloroaurate	deicide
amarillite	booty	chlorometry	depilatory
ambitty	bosselated	chylous	diabetic
amputee	branchiostegous	cimicoid	diacaustic
anastomose	braze	claustration	differential
ancred	brucine	cockade	dilatator
anemoscope	cacology	confiscable	dissection
anteriority	caliver	coranto	elaeometer

GeoSpell French: Spelling Bee Words

epactal	glyptic	keno	mimetesite
epergne	gossoon	kenos	miscellany
epicurism	granat	kippage	moellon
epizooty	harlequinade	knisteneaux	momental
exon	harmoniphon	labourdin	monadism
fertilize	harmoniphone	lacertiform	mooch
feudality	harridan	lactation	morocain
fibration	historicity	lacustrine	moschatel
fideism	hogo	lapies	musketeer
fideist	humeral	limbiferous	naiant
fideistic	humic	locale	naivety
filigree	hyalithe	lophine	napoo
flagelliferous	hydroceramic	lori	nasality
fluidity	hygienic	loris	neologist
frangipani	implacement	lozen	neurotrope
fumarine	incandescence	lucivee	ninon
gabbard	incandescent	machinist	nodicorn
galeiform	inconscient	mantua	nolition
galligaskins	infantile	marquee	nominalist
gam	infinitude	mashie	normality
gangrenous	insatiability	metalleity	nowed
gazetteer	insurgence	meteorolite	onomastics
gemauve	interiority	metreme	oolite
genitality	isocheim	millime	oolitic
genty	jetteau	mimetene	parado

GeoSpell French: Spelling Bee Words

parcourse	prosector	saltpetrous	tallyho
parried	pseudologue	salutary	tamp
parry	rabato	salver	tamping
passacaglia	racism	savan	tamps
passado	racist	saveloy	tenace
pedagogist	radzimir	scrutoire	terry
pelmet	rampion	sebilla	theodicy
phantasmagoria	randannite	sejant	timenoguy
phantasmagory	rarefactive	sextain	tizeur
phenakistoscope	relativity	shallot	tody
picotee	reveille	shinnery	trehala
pisciculture	reveree	shoder	truffle
pleuritic	riffler	siffilate	vancourier
plonk	romeite	sinologist	vanjohn
polonese	rondure	sinology	vermouth
pompion	roundelay	sorcerer	vie
prematurity	salification	spodumene	xebec
presbyope	saloop	stannic	zodico
promoter	salop	stibiconite	zydeco

GeoSpell French: Spelling Bee Words

Words from Old French :

bordage	burulee	culvertage	vavasory
broigne	buruly	esbat	
burelly	corbin	porket	

Words from Lousiana-French:

batture	cabree	gaspergou	perique
bayou	copalm	goujon	pulldoo
bogue	etouffee	grasset	sacalait
branchier	etouffees	jambalaya	tignon

GeoSpell French: Spelling Bee Words

French Phrases:

a cheval	avant-garde	café au lait	coup de foudre
a corps perdu	ballon d'essai	café brulot	coup de grace
a jour	basse-cour	café chantant	coup de main
a la	beau geste	café crème	coup de poing
a la carte	beaux arts	café filtre	coup de repos
a la mode	bel espirit	café noir	coup de theatre
a terre	bel etage	carte blanche	coup d'etat
aide-de-camp	belle epoque	carte de visite	coup d'oeil
aide-memoire	bete noire	carton pierre	coupe de ville
ailes de pigeon	blanc fixe	cause celebre	crème brulee
allee couverte	bois blanc	chaise longue	crème de moka
amour propre	bois cotelet	charge d'affaires	creme fraiche
ancien regime	bon mot	chef d'oeuvre	crepe suzette
arriere-ban	bon ton	chemin de fer	cul-de-four
arriere-pensee	bon vivant	cher maitre	cul-de-lampe
art nouveau	bon viveur	chose jugee	cul-de-sac
au courant	bon voyage	cinema verite	de rigueur
au fait	bouche fermee	clair de lune	de son tort
au gratin	brelan carre	comme il faut	de trop
au jus	brise vole	contre basse	déjà vu
au naturel	brun dore	contre viole	demi-sec
au pair	cache-peigne	contre-jour	dene
avant-corps	cachou de laval	cordon bleu	dernier cri
avant-courier	café au kirsch	cordon sanitaire	dernier ressort

GeoSpell French: Spelling Bee Words

droit du seigneur	faute de mieux	jeu d'esprit	opera bouffe
du jour	femme fatale	jeune fille	ouled nail
eau de cologne	fete champetre	jeunesse doree	papier mache
eau de javelle	feuille morte	joie de vi·vre	par excellence
eau de toilette	fievre boutonneuse	joie de vivre	parc ferme
eau-de-vie	film noir	laissez-passer	pas de basque
elan vital	fleur du mal	lese majeste	pas de bourree
eminence grise	fleur-de-lis	Louis Quatorze	pas de chat
en bloc	foie gras	Louis Quinze	pas de cheval
en arriere	folie a deux	main droite	pas de deux
en banc	force majeure	maniere criblee	pas de trois
en carre	gaude lake	maniere noire	pas-d'ane
en garde	grand choeur	mardi gras	passe-partout
en passant	grand guignol	menage a trois	passe-passe
en pointe	grand prix	menus plaisirs	pate brisee
en route	grande dame	mise-en-scene	peche melba
en tournant	haute couture	mise-en-table	petite sirah
enfant terrible	haute couture	nez perce	pied-a-terre
ente en point	haute ecole	nom de guerre	pince-nez
entre nous	haute monde	nom de plume	pis aller
esprit de corps	hors concours	nouveau riche	plat du jour
fait accompli	hors de combat	nouvelle vague	point d'angleterre
famille jaune	hors d'oeuvre	objet d'art	point d'appui
famille noire	idee fixe	objet trouve	
famille verte	je ne sais quoi	ombres chinoises	

GeoSpell French: Spelling Bee Words

point d'espagne	pot-au-few	saphir d'eau	toile de jouy
point d'esprit	pret-a-porter	savoir faire	tour de force
point d'hongrie	prie-dieu	savoir vivre	trompe l'oeil
poisson bleu	prix fixe	societe anonyme	vers de societe
port cochere	raison d'etre	soi-disant	vis-à-vis
port du salut	ranz des vaches	succes de scandale	volte-face
port salut	rime riche	succes fou	
porte cochere	robe de chambre	tete-a-tete	
poste restant	roman a clef	tete-beche	

GeoSpell French: Spelling Bee Words

GeoSpell French: Spelling Bee Words

References:

- Merriam Webster's Unabridged Dictionary – 3rd Edition
- How to Spell Like a Champ by Barry Trinkle, Carolyn Andrews, and Paige Kimble
- www.spellingbee.com
- www.wikipedia.com
- www.myspellit.com
- www.southasianspellingbee.com
- www.northsouth.org

Made in the USA
Monee, IL
01 February 2021